Books by Leza Lowitz

POETRY

America and Other Poems by Ayukawa Nobuo (cotranslator with Shogo Oketani, 2007)

Yoga Poems: Lines to Unfold By (2006)

100 Aspects of the Moon: Poems (2003)

Old Ways to Fold New Paper: Poems (1997)

FICTION

Green Tea to Go: Stories from Tokyo (2006)

NONFICTION

Sacred Sanskrit Words: For Yoga, Chant, and Meditation (with Reema Datta, 2006)

The Japan Journals, 1947–2004 by Donald Richie (editor, 2005)

Designing with Kanji: Japanese Character Motifs for Surface, Skin & Spirit (with Shogo Oketani, 2004)

Beautiful Japan: A Souvenir (1996)

ANTHOLOGIES

Manoa Journal: Silence to Light: Japan and the Shadows of War (editor, 2001)

Manoa Journal: Towards A Literature of the Periphery (editor, 1988)

A Long Rainy Season (editor, cotranslator with Miyuki Aoyama, 1995)

Other Side River (editor, cotranslator with Miyuki Aoyama and Akemi Tomioka, 1995)

Japan: Spirit and Form by Shuichi Kato (cotranslator with Junko Abe, 1994)

Yoga Heart

LINES ON THE SIX
PERFECTIONS

Yoga Heart

LINES ON THE SIX
PERFECTIONS

Leza Lowitz

with illustrations by Akiko Tanimoto

Stone Bridge Press • Berkeley, California

Published by
Stone Bridge Press
P. O. Box 8208, Berkeley, CA 94707
TEL 510-524-8732 • sbp@stonebridge.com • www.stonebridge.com

Printed in the United States of America.

10 9 8 7 6 5 4 3 2 1   2015 2014 2013 2012 2011

LIBRARY OF CONGRESS CATALOGING-IN-PUBLICATION DATA

Lowitz, Leza.
  Yoga heart : lines on the six perfections / Leza Lowitz ; with
illustrations by Akiko Tanimoto.
      p. cm.
  Includes bibliographical references.
  ISBN 978-1-933330-93-8
  1. Yoga—Poetry. I. Title.
  PS3562.O8963Y637 2011
  811'.54—dc21

                            2011018097

CONTENTS

K*shanti* P*aramita*
PATIENCE

V*irya* P*aramita*
JOYFUL EFFORT

Dhyana Paramita
STILLNESS

Prajna Paramita
WISDOM

for my beloved teacher

People sometimes ask writers, "Why did you write that book?" and the answer is often, "The book wrote me." For me, this has never been truer than with *Yoga Heart*, in which both the writing and the theme (the Six Perfections) *became* my daily practice. I wrote it because I had to learn what I was trying to live.

My previous book of poems, *Yoga Poems: Lines to Unfold By*. was structured around the eight limbs of yoga practice (Raja Yoga), which was a springboard for a personal and artistic inquiry into the physical, philosophical, and spiritual dimensions of yoga and life. With time and a deepening of practice, my exploration of yoga postures moved to the meditative aspects of yoga, and like many others, I sought to embrace a quieter, more inward-focused life. Paradoxically, as my attention turned inward, it turned outward to my community and my responsibility to live more peaceably, to serve others, and to try not to harm the planet.

But understanding isn't born overnight. My journey started over thirty years ago, when my teacher at Berkeley High School introduced our social studies class to the practice of Zazen meditation. I remember sitting in my hard wooden seat with my legs folded underneath me, trying to keep my back straight, eyes half-closed, fingers sealed in some mysterious mudra, and to watch my thoughts pass "like clouds in the sky." It was a lot to do at once. If I didn't find an immediate peace and stillness that took me far from teenage angst and delinquency, then at least I felt sufficiently intrigued to want to try again.

A few years later, as a student of karate, I chanted the *Heart Sutra*, dropping into the deep resonance of the words, though I didn't know their meaning. I started to write poems, sit in meditation, and practice Tai Chi, all to calm my mind. I studied Tibetan Buddhism at U.C. Berkeley, inspired (and intimidated) by the lengthy vows (eighteen root and forty-six secondary) that Mahayana disciples took to release themselves from the cycles of karma (*samsara*) and dedicate their lives to attaining enlightenment (*nirvana*) so that they could help others on the Bodhisattva path. Though I knew I'd probably never go to live in a monastery, I began to try to practice what Charlotte Jocko Beck calls "Everyday Zen." That meant sitting in meditation, and when not "sitting," attempting to see the world not through the mind and thoughts (theory and intellect) but through experience (sensation and essence), through what Buddhists call "no conceptual awareness," a meditative state of receptivity, and trying to become a better person. I saw how meditation opened a window into the possibilities that arose when my body, mind, and spirit were less fragmented but more integrated, and I actually started to feel connected to others rather than separate and lonely.

Instead of experiencing the world through a filter of habits and conditioning, I started to sense the vibrancy of what was in front of me, moment to moment, a bit more free of the veil of conditioning. Eventually, no longer addicted to the drama of struggle, I learned to let go and step out of my own way. The next step was seeing my life as a gift and trying to find ways to use the good fortune I'd been given to live in a land of plenty and peace, to help others whenever and however I could.

Beginning with "The Book"

As I continued to practice yoga, I saw that I'd been running away from myself through busyness, hiding from myself by throwing myself into work. I had to look deeply within and see the shadow parts of myself that I didn't like and needed to change. I allowed myself to physically break down and realize how much fear, anger, sadness, despair, and loneliness I had inside me. Yoga taught me in a direct way that we all share these things and are all connected in the desire to be happy and free of suffering. Yoga taught me how to change myself and to forgive myself and others. Actually it didn't even have to "teach" me; a transformation happened naturally through the practice. This is the beauty of working with the Outer Method (*asana*, *pranayama*) and the Inner Method (*dhyana*, or meditation).

I began to teach out of my house on the Northern California coast. I loved teaching and loved studying yoga.

So in 2003, when my husband decided it was time to move back to Japan after nine years in America, I told him the only way I felt I could keep my sanity in Tokyo was if I could do yoga there. But there were few studios, and though I could understand Japanese, I knew I would miss a lot not being taught in English.

Then I remembered: When I had gone on a yoga retreat in Haiku, Hawaii, in 2001 a powerful voice came to me and said, "You should move to Tokyo and open a yoga studio." I laughed at the time, as I had no plans to return to Japan. Was it Pele, the fierce Hawaiian Goddess, speaking? Or was it my own inner voice, trying to be heard? The benefits I received from yoga outweighed anything else I had received in life so far, so it made sense to share my love of yoga with others and give them this gift if I could. I decided to open a yoga studio in Japan.

Opening a studio in a foreign country was daunting, but I didn't think about all the things I couldn't do. Taking one step at a time, I felt guided to move forward even when things were challenging. Many wonderful people appeared to help make it happen. We found an empty room in an older building, and an architect friend contributed his designs. My husband helped me with the many logistics of starting a business in Japan. MC Yogi and Amanda designed my website and my logo. And so, Sun and Moon Yoga in Tokyo was born. It was an act of faith, a leap into the unknown, and a risk, but I decided

I'd rather risk failure by trying than sit around waiting for something to happen *to* me.

In California, we'd been surrounded by the sea and the mountains and open space and greenery. In Tokyo, there's not much green outside of a cup of tea. I wanted to make the studio green, calm, and feminine, with a round-shaped moon-viewing window. I wanted to offer a small oasis where people could discover and be their authentic selves.

This disconnect from others, from our deepest selves, and from nature is the cause of so many of our problems. The psychological costs are enormous—we smoke, drink, overeat, and overconsume, and we harm ourselves and others with little consciousness of the damage we are doing to ourselves, the animal world, and the environment. Many of us are missing a connection with others. What's the best way to reduce stress? Laugh. Hold someone's hand. But if your daily life consists of working nine to five (or even nine to nine like in Tokyo), when do you have a chance to connect with people? And if you don't connect first with yourself, how can you connect with others? This is a great gift that yoga offers—a *sangha*, a community. This community is beyond languages, countries, or borders.

Yoga helps us make that connection. We all know that yoga means "union"; union with our "higher self" and the divine, as well as recognizing and honoring that divinity within others. And it's essential now that we explore the other yogic values beyond the physical practice of *asana*. Interconnectedness is about giving and replenishing, not just receiving.

To this end, I wanted to use my thoughts, meditation, and yoga practice to change myself for the better, and to direct my energy toward helping others. But I didn't want to be a hypocrite or an evangelist. As charted in *Yoga Poems: Lines to Unfold By*, I tried to follow the eight limbs of yoga practice in my everyday life, attempting not to harm other beings and to live with honesty, generosity, and compassion. Over the years, I often failed, was lazy, or simply forgot how.

Then, in 2008, Ted Lafferty and other teachers from the Yoga Studies Institute visited Japan and taught Tibetan Heart Yoga at Sun and Moon. In simple yet powerful terms, they suggested that everything in the world was pure potential (emptiness) and explained how the world we experience might be a direct result of the seeds we've planted in our lives (karma), or possibly past incarnations. Their presence and teachings inspired me to start the practice of keeping "The Book"—a daily journal recording my thoughts, deeds, and words, allowing me to see how I am living my commitment to my "vows." Six times a day, I try to record my actions, words, and thoughts in six categories that parallel the *yamas* of the Eight Limbs of Yoga: protecting life (non-violence), honoring others' property (non-stealing), sexual purity (refraining from sexual misconduct), truthfulness (refraining from lying), speaking in ways to bring others together (refraining from divisive speech), and speaking gently (refraining from harsh words).

If I really wanted to live my yoga, I soon realized, I had to bring it to every word and deed, no matter how small. "The Book," Geshe Michael Roach says, is the secret to happiness and living one's dreams. By watching my ethics so closely, I'm attempting to live my yoga, or at least become much more aware of how I am in the world. If you want to change the world, the saying goes, change yourself. What better way to do this than starting with awareness of your actions, followed by taking responsibility for your actions, then changing those actions that don't align with a greater good? But this is not so easily done! Six times a day, writing down my deeds, words, and thoughts allows me to make a concerted effort to "walk my talk"— or notice and own up to it when I'm not. It has changed my life. Why? Because the quality of our thoughts determines the nature of our habits. Put simply: If I watch my thoughts closely I'll probably see some things that I don't like and want to change. In this way, my speech and deeds (habits) will change in a positive direction, and I can plant positive seeds for future actions to occur. I can work from the inside to affect the outside.

Through the power of keeping "The Book," twenty-five years after sitting in that classroom at U.C. Berkeley, I was led to reconnect with the six *paramitas* of Mahayana

Buddhism from the Lotus Sutra. These "Six Perfections" are innate human qualities that form a blueprint for living a virtuous life and transcending one's karma. They remind us that when we are born into this world, we join a web of interconnectedness with our fellow creatures, nature, the ecosystem, and the atmosphere. These treasures are:

Dana Paramita	Giving/Generosity
Shila Paramita	Kindness
Kshanti Paramita	Patience
Virya Paramita	Joyful Effort
Dhyana Paramita	Stillness
Prajna Paramita	Wisdom

They are called perfections because we are constantly led to practice these virtues until we "perfect" our human lives. Traditionally, the six treasures are cultivated by Bodhisattvas, enlightened beings who vow to help others attain enlightenment and keep doing so until all beings everywhere are free from suffering. Each perfection builds on another.

Awakening the Yoga Heart

The six *paramitas* form the underlying structure of this book. In the writing of these poems, my practice was to inquire: What does it mean to be generous—to give time, energy, money, resources, praise, attention, support, love?

What does it mean to receive? Can we accept generosity graciously and humbly?

As for kindness, how can we be truly kind to others and to ourselves? Another translation of the second perfection, *Shila Paramita*, is "ethics" or "morality." This means watching your thoughts, words, and deeds vigorously.

How do we cultivate patience? Geshe Michael Roach beautifully defines patience as a lack of anger. Can we catch ourselves before we react in anger to a challenging situation? Can we take a deep breath instead and see the person in front of us as no different from ourselves, indeed, as one? That's patience. Of course, patience is also slowing down, taking time to wait, being okay with not knowing what will happen next, even enjoying a liminal state where anything can arise.

And what of joy? Can we discover true joy—not by consuming, possessing, or achieving, but simply by honoring the beauty and richness of the moment, feeling contentment and satisfaction with things as they are, no matter how imperfect? Can we approach our daily work with true joy and passion, no matter how humble or tiring?

Then what of stillness? Can we embrace the stillness, just *being* rather than constantly *doing*? Can we allow time for prayer, meditation, being in nature, being alone with our own thoughts?

And what is wisdom? How do we come to understand the concept of emptiness and potentiality, and how can it help us live a better life? Can we see our neighbor as ourselves, the world and everyone in it as truly One? Can we see that the labels we attach to what we experience come from ourselves, and can we change the labels? Can we see our world and everything in it as nothing less than miraculous and divine? And what happens when something comes to knock us off-center, testing our faith? The Great East Japan Earthquake of March 2011 did just that. But we kept our doors open, and took refuge in our community and practice more than ever before.

These sixty poems were my attempt to hold onto this worldview, written over years of "Everyday Zen" practice, inspired by nature, yoga, meditation, scriptural study, Zen poetry, Buddhism, Osho, Tibetan Buddhism, Tibetan Heart Yoga, Tantra, ancient Japanese and Chinese poetry, Eastern philosophy, Western philosophy, Rumi, Kabir, sacred world poetry, haiku, love, and life. In them, I tried to keep the language simple and from the heart. In ways both literal and figurative, prescriptive and experimental, they seek to chart a journey from the physical body to the subtle body to the light body to bliss.

The stages to enlightenment are explained beautifully in *Lam Tso Nam Sum* (The Three Principal Paths). Its author, Tsongkapa Lobsang Drakpa (1357–1419), or Je Tsongkapa, lists the three steps (*Lam Rim*) to enlightenment. They are (1) Renunciation (ceasing looking for satisfaction in external things), (2) *Bodhichitta* (the wish to become enlightened for the benefit of all beings), and (3) the Wisdom of Emptiness (knowing that all things are pure potential; empty). These practices can take lifetimes, but simply being committed to living with the consciousness of inter-connectedness and to taking compassionate action can transform one's life forever. As my teacher explained, the prophecy "heaven is at hand" from *The Gospels of Thomas* is not an apocalyptic vision, but a view that "heaven" can exist here on earth by seeing the sacred in your world and making the world a better place for others if you have the eyes to see and the ears to hear it as such.

The best we can do is seek happiness so we can help others find happiness. These poems are a record of my attempt to do that, and an offering to my teachers and all those on the path. May they inspire your own awakened heart to continue to blossom and open to the joy of life, and may all beings everywhere be happy and free.

Offering
With grateful acknowledgment to my husband and best teacher, Shogo Oketani, whose calm presence and unconditional love and support have allowed me to grow and thrive for nearly two decades; to our beautiful son, Yuto Dashiell Oketani, who embodies freedom and bliss; to my kind and generous teachers Geshe Michael Roach, Lama Christie McNally, Ted Lafferty, Kimberley Theresa,

Narayani, MC Yogi & Amanda Giacomini, Yvonne Jaques, Venerable Lobsang Nyingpo, Mercedes Bahleda, Jill Edwards Minye, Veera Wibaux, Ganga White, Tracey Rich, Simon Simone, Lama Marut, Lama Winston McCullough, Clive Mayhew and Eriko Kinoshita, and all the translators at ACI. To my first meditation teacher Doug Powers, my first karate teacher Dardounian-sensei, my friends and co-creators of the magic at Sun and Moon Yoga—especially Em and Phil Bettinger, and Tomoko Kawahara, and all the wonderful teachers and souls who practice there, to John and Fran Lowitz and Donna and Dave Mendelsohn, my sisters Robin and Leslie and their families, and my entire family for support and love. To Aska, may you dance with a million coyotes and ninja-dogs in Nirvana.

Special thanks to dear friends Richard Ruben, Abigail Davidson, Maud Winchester, Lucas Reiner, Daissy Farias-Koch, Ralph Koch, Eric Gower, Edgar Honetschläger, Brian Bentley, Huntington Sharp, and Mihoko and Reiko Sugiura for "having my back" over the years. Publisher Peter Goodman of Stone Bridge Press deserves more thanks than I have words for, for giving me so many rich opportunities to learn, grow, and explore. The invaluable assistance of Linda Ronan, Nina Wegner, Noriko Yasui, and Jeanne Platt in making this book a reality is hugely appreciated. Deni Béchard became a last-minute savior, and Akiko Tanimoto delighted me with her beautiful calligraphy born from years of dedicated yoga practice—what a revelation. Christopher Yohmei Blasdel made these words dance in the air with his masterful shakuhachi. Joe Zanghi, as always, has offered greatly valued support. A million kisses to the Tarakas for being the best siblings one could ever want. Special appreciation to Jack Kornfield for the beautiful lectures, "Your Buddha Nature: Teachings on the Ten Perfections."

Heartfelt gratitude to the publishers of the following magazines, websites, and anthologies where these poems appeared, sometimes in different form: *Tundra* ("On Modesty"), *Oakland Out Loud* ("On Modesty"), *The New American Imagist* ("On Modesty," "Why I Love Rock Gardens," "The Room"), *The Tokyo Advocate* ("Waiting," "Compassion"), *If Women Ruled the World*/Inner Ocean Publishing ("Waiting"), *The Poetry of Yoga* ("In a Corner of the Body, a Thief Sits Waiting"), *Poems of Awakening* ("Waiting"), Poetry Nippon ("Like Water," "Space-Time Cowboy," "Two As One," "The Tiger," "The Flame").

To all, this book is offered with love and joy.

Leza Lowitz
Tokyo, Japan

All author proceeds from the sale of the book will go to relief efforts to people and animals affected by the Great East Japan Earthquake of March 11, 2011.

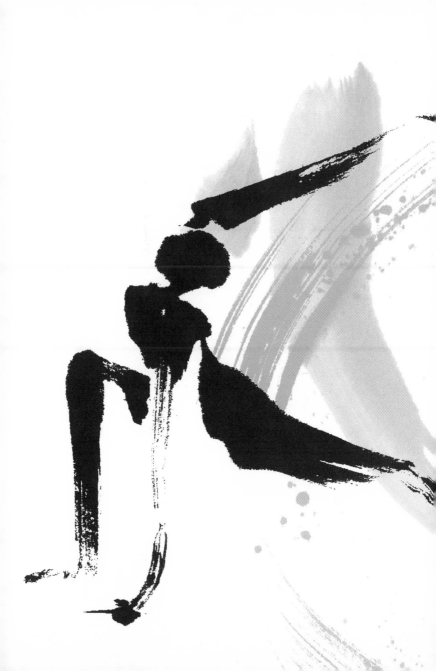

Dana Paramita

GIVING

Like Water

Be like the river—
flowing.
Be like the lake—
calm.
Be like the ocean—
roar.
Be like the dam—
restrained.
Be like the waterfall—
tumbling.
Be like the rain—
pour.
Be like ice—
solid.
Give like water—
naturally,
assuming
right form.

Bamboo

Everything known was once unknown.
Everything grown was once ungrown.

Strong roots of bamboo,
supporting the earth beneath,
holding the branches above—
this web of being.

Yielding to the sky,
rooted to the earth.
The path
between ground and sky
unshakeable.

In this way,
what you touch
touches you.

Tonglen

"We all have the seeds of violence within us," said the
    Dalai Lama.
"We all have the seeds of peace."

War and peace—
in the law of dharma
one can't exist
without the other.

In the awakened heart,
honor and nation
enemy and border
dissolve.

Whether in violence,
whether in peace,
what we give
is what we receive.

When I hurt you,
I hurt myself.
When I love you,
I love myself.

Generosity

Generosity
is the sun—
white star
of warmth and light—

shining
on and
on.

Never asked,
never
asking.

Accepting
nothing
in return.

In Praise of Wildness

> *"Wildness is the state of complete awareness. That's*
> *why we need it."*
> —*Gary Snyder,* Turtle Island

The more still we become
the more wildness arises within.

Does a lion feel the pleasure
of its power gathering
like river water at a dam,
its strength building as it sleeps,
dreaming of the chase?

Can a snake never be straight,
but merely uncoiled,
waiting to spring to movement?

Is a hurricane a wilderness of air?
A cyclone a suspended door
to a turbulent sky?

Does the heart grow larger
in the glassed-in chest
when we forgive?

That's the wildness.
Can you let it
embolden you,
made form, made flesh?

From this wildness,
can every cell in your body
find gratitude,
make praise?

Devotion

Long days of study,
taking a sledgehammer
to the habits of the mind.
Crushing thoughts of you and me,
I me mine
with a thousand steadfast blows.
Who dares intervene
between the iron
and the flesh?

To learn the scriptures
is to take up the hammer.
To live the scriptures
is to dissolve the Self
into the blows.

Forged on the anvil,
your voice could sing
a hundred holy chants
or praise the beauty
of the single song to the Divine
and it would be the same.

Sing, even if to yourself,
even if no one is listening,
and in the singing,
allow your heart
to finally be heard.

Know Your Seasons

If you wish
to become
natural,
know your seasons.

When you rain,
submerge.
In wind and snow,
howl and freeze.

In your fire,
purify and die.
Find repose in ice.

Don't lie to yourself.
Go with the changes,
and the body will not stray,
the heart will never contract.

It is enough
"to know that this
passing is all . . ."

Shattered

Giving is living.
Giving is letting go.

What we hold onto
holds us back.
What we release
allows us to fly.

This simple lesson
takes a lifetime to learn,
yet once learned
is never forgotten.

Like a glimpse of our true nature,
our Buddha nature
in the mirror,
it shatters us.

Naikan

A woman walks into
the door to her life,
banging her head against it
for the hundredth time,
seeing nothing but darkness.

She knows there must be light.
How else has she been growing
in that dark corner for so many years?

Starting with her life,
she reflects on the many things
she's been given.
How could she not feel abundant?
How could she not love her mother?

Without blame or regret,
humbled by those who cared for her
(those she troubled, inconvenienced, angered,
hurt, abused, or worse, ignored)
she takes the door from its hinges
and steps outside.

To her surprise, she doesn't lose herself
or fall to pieces.
Rather, she grows light
like the clouds, lifted by those who carried her.

Transformed by this simple shift to gratitude
she vows to be truly satisfied with what she has—
to make of her life a gift,
to stand naked before the world and serve.

Prasad

—for my Lama

That sound you hear?
It's my frozen heart melting.

Bringing each drop to my lips,
I cover my body freely,

wet with your name.
My lips become your lips,

my body your body.
When I take you into me,

the world goes
on forever.

I will
find peace

in these
fragments.

This pain
will be the cure.

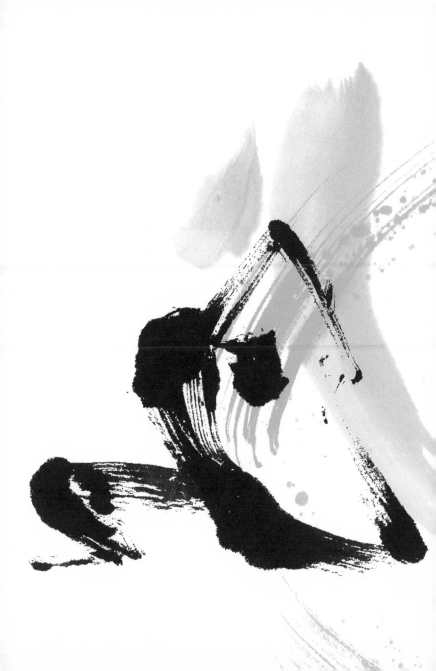

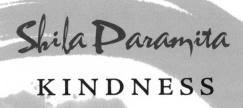

Shila Paramita

KINDNESS

Space-Time Cowboy

Eyes roving the landscape,
blazing through the horizon
in search of another conquest
lost in a thousand dry dust storms,
mocked by tumbleweeds, the sudden rattle of snakes.

Your cowboy duds have dried to rawhide ropes.
You've fought so long you no longer know
who fires the bullets or where to aim.
You thought you'd won all your battles
but the wind is an army of hungry ghosts
marching across the desert,
crying bullets of rain into your chest.
The evening light tilts like a curtain
drawn over the insatiable plains.

When you finally come to the duel
your gun is empty, your draw is a blank.
Nothing to do now but unsaddle yourself
and ride the plains of the heart.

Let kindness run roughshod over past and future.
Let yourself be completely undone

in the place where rider and horse,
land and sky, heaven and earth are one.

Why be just a cowboy?
Why be just a prairie?

Be every dry desert,
every high mountain,
every low-slung valley,
every raging river,
every two-bit ghost town,
every abandoned train track.
Walk softly over every possible landscape you can
     imagine
in this vast, majestic world.

The Choice

Look not at the faults of others,
at what they have done or left undone.
Rather look at what you yourself
have done or left undone.
—Dhammapada, *Verse 50*

Get off the train of criticism,
or stay where you are if you must—
stuck on the tracks,
blocking your own journey.

You can blame others endlessly
or take responsibility, right now,
for yourself.
Be neither victim nor vanquisher.
Let your failures humble you.
Humility breeds gratitude,
which gives birth to compassion.

This is *moksha*,
liberation.
The ability to see the choice,
then make the choice.

Choose Wisely

I've never been to the rainforest,
but I can wrap myself in blankets of imagined moss
and be consoled by the deepest green.

I've never met my ancestors
but I can see them in my dreams,
vivid as the cobblestone streets they walked on
taking only what they could carry.

You've never seen your future self,
yet you can create her in each moment
through your thoughts, words, and deeds.

We don't live alone.
We won't die alone.

Don't forget this.
Never forget this.

Choose wisely, choose well.
Just don't be afraid to choose.
Then stand firmly by your choice.

The Edge

Each time the world
pushes you to the edge
asking of you
more than you can bear,
go ahead anyway
even if—or because—
you're straining against
an invisible net.

Let yourself burst at the seams
until the seams themselves stretch,
and the net tears, floats away
into the nothingness
from which you came.
Who holds the net anyway?

Everything it contains
will come rushing forth.
Embrace it all, and then some.
Watch yourself.
Don't just sit on your mat and dream.
Change yourself one thought at a time.
Give love to others.
You'll grow bigger than you ever imagined.

So much I want to say to you, teacher!
But you say: *Just live your best life.*
It speaks so much more eloquently
than words.
To my teacher then,
I give it all.

Rock Gardens

There are those who believe life is like a recalcitrant
        garden—
no matter how many times you pull the weeds,
they'll grow right back: no provocation, no fertilizer,
barely any sunshine, not even much water.
They think that like the poison Oleander
the more you abuse yourself, the stronger you grow.

I'm not a believer.
Drench your neighbor in compassion,
give them a Japanese rock garden any day.
They don't care to be cultivated by abrasion,
don't want to blossom under duress.
They need only to be tended to gently,
contemplated in serenity by moonlight,
raked over gently,
revered.

Just Be

Inside the body,
the sound
of rain falling.
Outside the body,
rain falling.

In the gap,
all things die
and are reborn.

Between in-breath
and out-breath
an endless pilgrimage
to Being.

Today,
be thankful
for this
liminal space.
In it you'll find
a perfect home.

The Magpie

The heart is an enormous palace.
Not always glittering,
it too needs to be cleaned.
Every day,
throw open its doors—
welcome beggar, thief, fool, saint,
sunlight and storm,
even the dark clouds of night
that fall over it.

Invite the wrathful demons
to feed unabashedly on your afflictions:
jealousy, pride, stinginess, anger, impatience, fear.

For when the darkness breaks the light is brighter,
and in the dawn
after you've seen yourself clearly—
you'll know what power there is in clarity.
How easy it will be,
then, to fly like the magpie
straight and fearlessly
into all that dazzles—
all that loves
and is beloved.

Earth Household

There's a place in the heart
where the divine spirit lives.
Inhale and the light expands within.
Exhale and it radiates
covering the earth,
lighting the path.

Release yourself
from the same old patterns,
limits, and thoughts,
fall into joy
and start again
where you are.

Having given all of yourself
and made a home of yourself,
now you can make a home for others.

Ask yourself honestly:
What do you hunger for?
You will answer:
To be fed, surely,
but mainly to nourish.

Resistance

Not words
but the echo

of a temple bell
after it has been struck.

Not action
but true awareness.

Form finds form
as in painting, prayer, song.

Resistance too,
finds a welcome,

for without resistance
there is no yielding,

without struggle
no triumph,

without sound,
no silence.

What if all your mistakes
were really divine designs

to teach you how to see
beyond yourself?

What you struggle against
eventually becomes you,

the way river becomes ocean,
small water inseparable

from big water,
everything in flow.

Compassion

She took her time
turning her fork in the flesh
of the big winter fish, tearing
at its face—
coruscant gray,
eye turned up—
like a small moon
on a celadon plate.

At the elegant country *ryokan*
tucked into Kyoto's northern hills,
she ate the fish slowly
afraid of bones.
And then she caught the glint
of a fishhook
bent tightly into its cheek,
and she vanished
into the river,
feeling the cold rush
swim against her skin,
the bump of rock and glide of current
the freedom of floating,
the way all good journeys begin.

Unsatisfied by the smart conversation
at the table:
a new war in a far-off country,

books read or unread,
difficult children or love affairs gone wrong . . .
all the usual talk on an outing
such as this . . .

She wished,
just this once,
that she'd placed
the fish's mouth
in her mouth
unthinkingly,
wished that she'd
suffered the hook,
felt exactly another's pain.

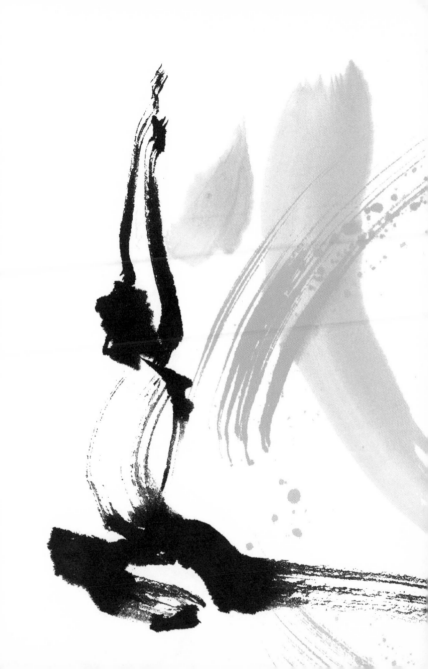

Kshanti Paramita
PATIENCE

What Does It Mean to Be Zen?

To do nothing?
Think nothing?
Be nothing?
Impossible.

To be Zen
is just to be yourself—
not name nor job nor history,
not likes nor dislikes,
thought or no-thought,
desire or despair.

But what is self?
Where does self reside?

(Hint: In what we do for others.)

Most difficult of all
is to meet yourself
where you are,
and abide there
completely
just as you are

accepting whatever arises
from moment to moment.

All else happens on its own accord.

Monkeymind Market

Like the best convenience store in the world,
the mind is always open.
Its job is to work non-stop,
offering a thought here,
a memory there,
attempting to sway you with a new plan
at the check-out counter,
an impulse buy you can't refuse.

Some purchase everything in sight,
desperate for satisfaction.
Some pick up each item,
turn it over endlessly
only to put it back down.
Some look for the best quality,
the limited edition,
others only for a bargain.
Some try to smash the shelves,
sending the products
tumbling to the ground.

So don't waste any more time!
Sort through the destruction
looking for fragments.

Just taking stock,
putting each thing in its place,
observing, then finally
discovering
the empty spaces
between aisles,
such fertile ground
to plant
all those
fragrant,
rich seeds.

Speak to Me

They say the Buddha's first words
after enlightenment
were a poem.

Entering the hermitage,
the poet travels deep into
the guest-house of the body.
Though the walls are thin
the floors are bare
the ceiling cracked
and the rain pours through,
here human nature
entwines with nature.

Speak gently.
Do not judge others harshly
lest you yourself be judged.
Choose your words wisely.
Hold your tongue when angry.

Just so, there's a circle in the ceiling
for viewing the moon,
a reflecting pool

of the sphere of the heart
empty and full.

What you say about others
returns in what is said about you.
The moon on the water,
becomes one with the water,
past nesting in future,
no need for more words.

Teabowl Zen

—for Japan, after the quake

Does beauty arise
from ash and ruin,
like the glaze of the teabowl
born from the fire?

You either build
or you destroy.
Turn toward the pain.
Let it sear into you.
Remember the harm
you have done to the earth.

Vow to repay the earth
for its kindness.
These scars will be
our path to compassion,
our mistakes
the road to a peaceful future
more valuable
than the purest gold.

On Modesty

He called himself the farmer of Katsushika,
and thirty other names, moving ninety-three times,
following the movement of seas, waterfalls, islands, the
     moon.
His father was a mirror polisher for the Shogun.
He captured Mt. Fuji from every perspective,
his eye like a fox, like a camera.
He wanted to live to ninety, but after making thirty
     thousand prints,
Hokusai died at eighty-nine, saying:
If heaven gives me even five more years, I shall
surely become a great artist.

Simplicity

Insight is the gift
of seeing reality as it is.
Not as it *was*,
nor as we wish it to be
but just this,
just *this*,
just *this*.

Go ahead and complicate things
if you like.
When you figure them out
another complication
will surely arise.

Why not simplify?
If you have the good fortune and leisure
to spend so much time in your head,
when you get off your cushion,
why not go out and be useful?

In this way,
without expectation or hope
without attachment or plans
stillness meets emptiness,

where wisdom arises.
There you'll find the whole
and enter it
as it
enters you.

Waiting

You keep waiting for something to happen,
the thing that lifts you out of yourself,

catapults you into doing all the things you've put off,
the great things you're meant to do in your life,

but somehow never quite get to.
You keep waiting for the planets to shift

the new moon to bring news,
the universe to align, something to give.

Meanwhile, the piles of papers, the laundry, the dishes,
        the job—
it all stacks up while you keep hoping

for some miracle to blast down upon you,
scattering the piles to the winds.

Sometimes you lie in bed, terrified of your life.
Sometimes you laugh at the privilege of waking.

But all the while, life goes on in its messy way.
And then you turn forty. Or fifty. Or sixty . . .

and some part of you realizes you are not alone
and you find signs of this in the animal kingdom—

when a snake sheds its skin, its eyes glaze over,
it slinks under a rock, not wanting to be touched,

and when a caterpillar turns to a butterfly
if the pupa is brushed, it will die—

and when the bird taps its beak hungrily against
        the egg
it's because the thing is too small, too small,

and it needs to break out.
And midlife walks you into that wisdom

that this is what transformation looks like—
the mess of it, the tapping at the walls of your life,

the yearning and writhing and pushing,
until one day, one day

you emerge from the wreck
embracing both the immense dawn

and the dusk of the body,
glistening, beautiful

just as you are.

Stop the Bullet

Lincoln resisted going to war,
against the "better angels of our nature."
And when the Civil War was over,
even the photos were discarded,
their glass plates sold to gardeners
for conservatory walls.
As the sun burned the images away,
hundreds of red roses
absorbed the light to grow.

Over a century and a half later,
an eighty-two-year-old surfer rides the waves,
recalls being strafed by machine-gun fire
on Pearl Harbor
as the planes flew low,
the red circle on the fuselage
etched in memory.

So many bodies, not enough caskets,
they had to put two men in each—
young American men along
with the Japanese pilots
who killed them.
Is there a better metaphor for war?

When the soldier arrives,
bleeding in the doorway,
can you recognize him as yourself
and let him in?
Once you let him in,
you'll meet many more like him.

Let him turn himself inside out
like a kimono—
black on the outside,
pattern on the inside—
the heart's hidden wounds exposed.
Let his sorrow intensify with each breath.
Let him live.

Turned inside out,
he will show you two kinds of hearts:
one that moves
and one that is frozen.

Do not temper outrage.
Do not try to craft perfection.
Only do what you have to do
to forgive.

The greater the battle,
the deeper the peace.

Released from the pull of separation,
go forth with the intention
to save your own life.

If you want to see peace in the world,
kill the anger within your own heart.

If you're still suffering,
if you still must live in the night sky,
seek to uplift others.
Do not live alone!

Remember—
even the stars
keep company
with the moon.

Against the Need to Know

It's difficult to enter
the silence that envelops everything.
Yet, to become truly yourself,
you must rebel against
the need to know.
Meditate and see yourself with diamond eyes—
strong, sharp, and clear.

Control nothing.
Learn each inch of yourself:
flesh, bone, blood, joy,
desire, despair.
Then know others as just the same.

What turns your body into light?
What turns your life into love?
Find it and use it.
Use it unabashedly,
recklessly, radically
with your total being.
Use your life for others.
Go on.
Use it.

And then,
in place of *why*,
true knowing arises.

Sadhana

—after Ho Sen

In summer,
the leaves of the Japanese maple
brighten in shades of green.

In autumn,
people travel from far-away towns
to see the blazing red glory.

In winter, the leaves
turn brown,
releasing into the earth.

Come spring,
they'll be carried
down the mountain

on the very same rains
that fed the buds
yet unborn within.

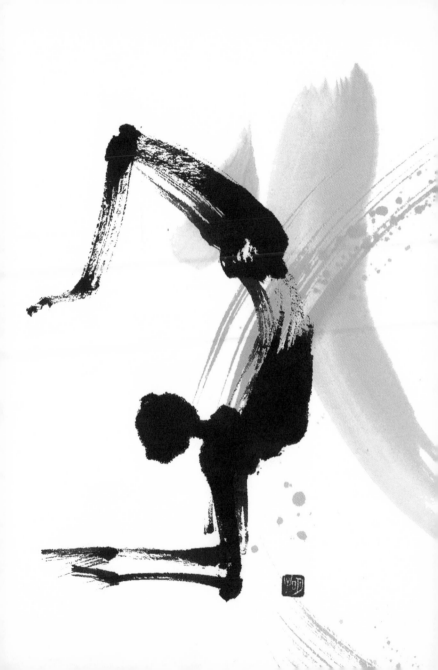

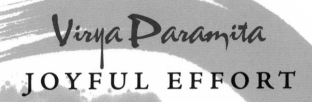

Virya Paramita
JOYFUL EFFORT

Shiva, Lord of the Dance

Root one foot into the earth.
Lift the other back like a bow,
taking aim straight ahead
to the heart of the soul's melody.
Let the foot beat a small crescendo
in the palm of the hand,
let the standing leg
ring out a bass note strong and clear.
Find balance amidst the clamor
of the world's many musics,
harmony rising from the ash
of Shiva's cosmic dance.

The curtain has risen.
This is your dance.

To destroy we must create.
To create we must believe.
Destruction and creation are the same, tied to each other.
So be an artist, create your perfect world.
This is the awakening.
There is no other way to know the dancer
than to surrender
to the dance.

Asana

If you had come easily
slip of joint into bone,
we might have missed you
for the teacher you are.

If you had simply arisen
from the body like a sigh
we might have completely
taken you for granted.

If you had come without effort
like a dream or sleep
we wouldn't have bothered
to learn your name.

But since you came like a warrior
engaging us in fierce battle
we want to know
every inch of you
so that when your power
arises in us,
it bears witness to the struggle,
lights up the stage for the
hero within.

Skydancer of Bliss

Do you die a little each day,
forgetting who you are?

When you forget,
as we all do,
get onto your yoga mat
or go out into nature and get quiet.

Start up your breath,
think good thoughts about others,
fit the shape of beauty
into each curve of your back,
worship the beautiful river of your spine,
bless it for keeping you alive.

Drench the ground you stand on
with the light of life.
Move your winds
from the left and the right sides
into the central channel,
into the arms of the Skydancer of Bliss.

Then watch those thirty-six vertebrae
become divine prayer wheels
spinning rapturously
with the sacred.

In a Corner of the Body,
a Thief Sits Waiting

In a corner of the body,
a thief sits waiting
to steal your affection.
Like a pickpocket in the black market,
he hides in the dark alleys of the body,
but your virtues are a lantern
rooting him out.

Catch a glimpse
as he rounds the corner
hoping to hide in the hip joint.
Watch him fly
as he darts between the shoulder blades,
wedges himself therein.
Marvel as he ducks
under the sacrum, sticks there
like a thumbtack.
Rejoice to see him tumble
headfirst into the pelvic bowl,
jeering as he peers around its rim.

Don't let his alacrity fool you.
He's as slow as what limits you,

holding you back just as much.
Once you catch him with your awareness,
don't throw him into prison.
Don't bind him up in rope.
Rather, hang him out in the light,
and praise him effusively.

For when the chase is over,
he will have taught you
the many secrets of the maze,
and you can start to polish
all those precious gems
he's been guarding.

Samurai Yogi

The samurai's sword
is alive with spirit,
each blade containing
a life-force of its own.

The yogi's body is the sword.
Enlivening the flesh with *prana*
awakening the mind through meditation,
cutting through illusion.

Enjoy your work.
No matter how
hard or humble,
work with joyful effort.

The samurai says:
It's a good day to die.

The yogi says:
It's a good day to live.

Sukha, Sthira

Steadiness and ease,
two dimensions of an *asana*,

like a tea bowl and tea.
Without the tea,

a bowl has no function.
Without the bowl,

the tea cannot find form.
Holding steady, we pour ourselves into the world.

Spirit pervades our lives
as clay pervades the teabowl.

The one who meditates without the view
is like a blind man wandering the plains.

The nature of the mind is no different
from the forms arising in it.

So polish the cup.
Be complete in filling, being filled.

Touching the Buddha, Touching the Mat

Sweep your hands in the air
as if across
a big fat Buddha,
touching wrist, chest, ankle, heart, knee—
where the body
has known pain,
or just no longer
wants to feel.

Place your hands
upon the mat
as if touching sacred earth.
Draw up healing light
into the central channel,
where union is your natural state.

Understand your mission.
Kill the pain body
once and for all.
Awaken the bliss body
through understanding karma
and emptiness,
by cultivating the wish
to help others.

Then,
so much love and wonder
rising,
arising
never to leave.

Gravy

When Ray Carver died
from a brain tumor caused by lung cancer—
having escaped death by alcohol a decade earlier—
his wife found a scrap of paper on his desk
near his typewriter.

Forgive me if I'm thrilled with the idea,
but just now I thought that every poem I write
ought to be called "Happiness."

No heroics. No apologies.
Just every day. Happiness.
Near the end of his life he wrote:
It was gravy. All gravy.

Let yourself say:
"Every poem will be called happiness."
"Every day will be devoted to helping others be happy."

Right

When
the
Buddha
died
he
lay
on
his
right
side,
deep
in
comfortable
rest.
Even
then,
in
his
final
moments,
fully
awake
to
sensation.

Lovers Count Laughter

Wise
men
count
blessings.

Fools
count
problems.

Lovers
count
laughter,
cherished
and
free.

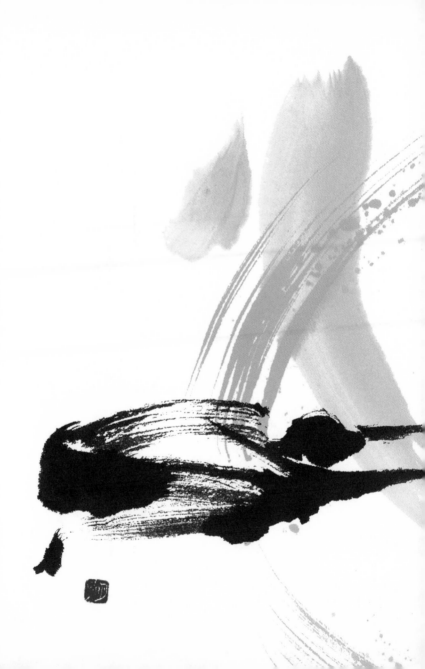

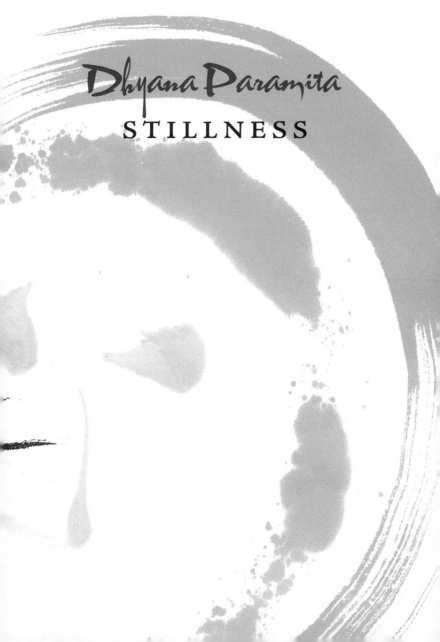

Dhyana Paramita

STILLNESS

Diamond Sutra

Purifying everything—
thoughts, words, deeds
in the fire,
polishing the carbon
to perfection.

Setting the rough stone
of your life
in wisdom,
creating a diamond
for the ages.

Eight-Bar Meditation

What you see in your world
is what you've created in your life.
You've heard it before:
If you want to see peace,
be gentle.
If you want to see beauty,
live gracefully.
If you want to have love,
give love.

Come back to yourself.
Again and again.
Let these virtues be your refuge.
From there it's easy:
Give. Serve. Love.

In the end,
there's only the path
and the
wayfarer on it.

Shanti, shanti, shantih.
Peace, peace, peace.

The Poem, The Body

Each newborn body
has an unwritten story upon it;
the mystic can see this.
Each white page
has an epic on it;
the poet can see this.

Where to start?
What to say?
Pick up the pencil,
take it across the page.
It will find its own tale.

Pick up your body,
carry it deeper into stillness.
It will find its dance.

Let yourself be written.
Let yourself be danced.
Overwrite if you must.
Dance to delirium.
But censor nothing,
not one single step,
not one single word.

Loss & Gain

In this life
we lose
nothing of value.

We'll never lose
what we've given away.

Nothing remains
that we can't find again
through selflessness
and compassion.

Of these riches,
we can never
be dispossessed.

Only the Dervish, Only the Dance

If you had one day left to live
how would you spin out
the story of your life?

Tangled in likes and dislikes,
locked in a perpetual dance with adversity,
there comes a day when you have to stop
"againsting" or you will die.

The day has come, my friend.
Let yourself die.

Tonight, you and the divine
can dance together
spinning into one another,
beside each other
beneath each other
above each other
below each other
inside each other
outside each other.

Shake your body free
so hard it divests itself

of attractions and aversions.
Purify yourself of pain
until there is no
you, no me, no *us*,
only ecstasy,
only the dance.

Thirty Skins

Thirty or forty skins, as thick
and hard as an ox's or a bear's,
cover the soul, Meister Eckhart said.
What's beneath the hardness?
What's piled under years of deceit,
selfishness, blame, apathy,
ambition, greed?

No wonder the skin is hard,
resistant to being pulled off.
No surprise it rivals
the strength of ox, of bear.
Stubborn armor of ego—
all that guarding, protecting!
On the path, this skin of ignorance
can either be shed
or ripped off.
We have the choice.

When we understand the nature of things
as they are—
the world inside
the world outside
are mere constructs—

the world we see before us
is what we've done to others.

Now is the time to strip away your selfishness.
Now is the time to be empowered.
Now is the time to let the heart be soft,
ready to give in,
like the parched ground
yielding to each drop
of precious rain.

One Hand Clapping

What
is the sound
of one
hand clapping?

Everything
clapping!

The Odyssey

On and on we row,
drifting this way and that
through the raging tempest
of hours, days, years.

Great sea of mind-waves!
Not wind nor rain
sun nor shadow
sound nor silence
intervenes.

What can stop this great wave of time?

Only love can lash itself to the mast—
love of self,
love of others,
love of every living being
truly cherished as one,
only love.

Spanda

Turn down the volume
of the world.
Turn up the sacred pulse,
ever-flowing beat of life,
rhythm of energy within.

Don't run after pleasure
or wallow in pain.
Refuse to be angry
even when someone comes
screaming in high volume at your face.
Try instead to help them.

Just to see the world this way
before *before*
after *later*
is a revelation.

Rest in the understanding
that the difficulties you experience
are old karmas ripening to be released,
surfacing to be purified.

This is your training ground
for cultivating *bodhichitta*—
the wish to become enlightened
to help others.

Welcome the unknown,
embrace the unknowable,
the way you greet your shadow
as it follows you unseen—
always there
in the movement
in the stillness,
taking its sweet time.

Grace

Perhaps a feeling of relief
washes over you
the way you unexpectedly
see the face of someone you love
in a crowd.

Maybe a prayer fills your heart
as you sit
in the midst of your crowded life,
welcoming the empty space.

This is your daily work.
To live this life
as if she's there
just over your shoulder,
an angel—
weightless in her wings
breaking open the sky
at your back.

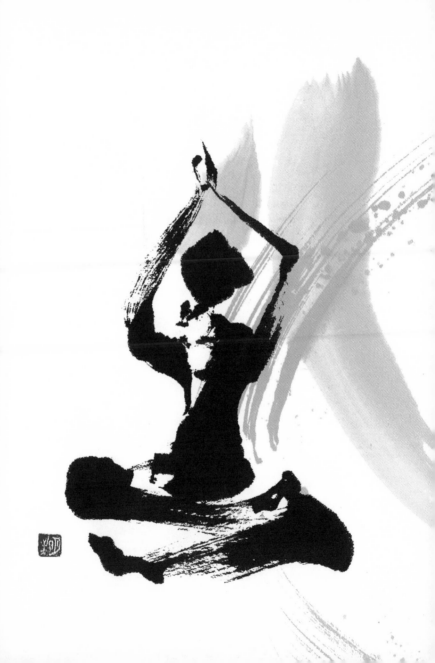

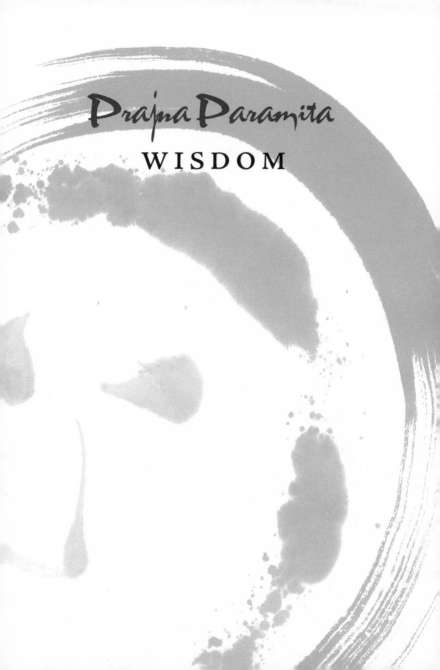

Prajna Paramita
WISDOM

Butterfly

An orange and black butterfly
alights on a potted sage.

So put one hand on top of the other,
spread your fingers into wings,
move them up and down,
together and apart.

What else is there to do
than to become the butterfly,
winging through the world,
enchanted?

Its freedom our freedom,
its beauty our beauty.

Karma Riddle #1

—for GMR/LCM

The flame depends
upon the wick.

When the wick burns up
the flame goes out.

What is the cause
of the wick burning?

The first place
the flame touches?

The last?

A point
in between?

You see?

The Tiger, The Flame

The tiger mauls me.
I am the tiger.
The fire burns me.
I am the fire.
The earth covers me.
I am the earth.
The wind envelops me.
I am the wind.
The water engulfs me.
I am the water.
The sun warms me.
I radiate.
The mirror shatters me.
I am the mirror.

My thoughts, deeds, actions—
these seeds,
and *only* these seeds
plant my life.

My rage leads me to the tiger.
My blindness sends me into fire.
My jealousy turns to earth.
My fear to wind.

My sadness releases to water,
My ignorance melts to sun.

Nothing exists on its own.
Let each unite and bless the other.

Ehipassiko
—*after Leonard Cohen*

coming/going
living/dying

open the gate
to yourself

blaze forth
with fearless love

yesterdaytodaytomorrow
forever and a day

the view beckons
even when your back is turned

So turn around!
Pay attention!

Notice cracks
in the smallest places,

rivers of light
shining through.

All Is Mother

The old white boat
and the crooked blue river—

the beauty I see
and the beauty I do—

one cannot exist
without the other.

That's why you must see
everyone you meet as your mother,

and vow to repay
her kindness.

Santosha

Praise to my hands,
for bringing food to my mouth.
Praise to my mouth, my stomach, my spleen.
Praise to the farmer, the soil, the seeds, the vegetables,
	the rain.
Praise to the truckers, the packers, the shippers, the
	sellers.
Praise to the cook.
Praise to the potter, the dishwasher.
Praise to my feet.
Praise to this body, a chariot
wending its way along the path.
Praise to the steps.
Praise to the passenger.
Praise to all who came before us,
guiding the way.
Praise to our teachers, our mothers, our fathers,
those who gave birth to us, raised us up.
Praise to the city.
Praise to the path.
Praise to the water.
Praise to the earth and the sky.
Praise to the song.
Praise to small things each day.

Invisible things—
recognized, honored, celebrated
become enormous.
Santosha. Contentment.
Praise to
waking up
to this.

Emptiness

Once I stole from others.
Soon, all I had disappeared.

Once I spoke ill of others.
Before long, no one listened to me.

Once I treated others carelessly.
My world spiraled into chaos.

Then my teacher appeared and set me on the path.

I saw the world clearly.
What I'd done to others

Was surely done unto me.
A million times imprinted in my mind.

I saw that all was empty,
and that empty was not void.

I saw that everything
was pure potential—

and that the nature of things
depended on where I stood.

What I thought solid
could in fact be fluid,

what I thought weapon
might be instead tool,

who I thought foe
could indeed be friend.

Once I saw that, I received more than
I ever imagined.

My own heart returned to me
begging to be forgiven.

Seeds

Each seed we plant
comes back to us,
bearing similar fruit.

What we plant flowers forth.
Why plant bitterness
when you can plant joy?

Why plant hatred
when you can plant love?
Why hold onto anything,
even this life?

Who wants to live forever?
Rather, let your life
ripen completely.

And when it's time to fall,
let it fall,
lush and full.

You'll live forever
in all
your good deeds.

Two As One

—after a priestess of Inanna (2000 BCE)

My lover, my heart.
Come to my bed.
Let us stand before each other,
the beauty of our two faces
seen clearly as one.

Strike my heart
with your body.
Sweet nectar of pleasure,
sweet song of pain.
Tell me all
and I will please you,
receive pleasure from you
completely.

Let us stand naked
before each other
clothed in the richness
of this world,
because I love you,
because you love me.

The Six Perfections

Be generous:
giving.
Be virtuous:
kind.
Be patient:
devoid of anger.
Be happy:
cherish others over yourself.
Be still:
honor the silence.
Be wise:
understand the nature of all things
as empty.

Rejoice in these six perfections.
They are
the path and the light
a meteor
an illumination
a shelter
a home
a goal
an island
a mother and a father.

The six perfections lead to knowledge,
to understanding,
to supreme, truly perfect enlightenment.

Practice the six perfections to perfection.
Then lavishly pass them on.

page 16   According to its website, the Yoga Studies In-
stitute is "a non-profit educational institute that
thoroughly grounds students in the classical tradi-
tion of yoga. The YSI program reunites the 'outer'
methods (working with the physical postures and
breath) with the the traditional 'inner' methods
(cultivating the ethical restraints and commit-
ments, meditation, and wisdom) into a powerful
synthesis the ancients called 'royal yoga'" (www.
yogastudiesinstitute.org).

page 17   To find more about "The Book," visit www.
world-view.org. You can download it for free
there. Keeping a daybook of your behavior is a
great practice to ensure that you're acting with
awareness. Many great figures throughout history,
including Benjamin Franklin, have done it.

page 18   The later *Ten Stages Sutra (Dasabhumika)* lists
another four perfections: *Upaya Paramita* (Skillful
Means), *Pranidhana Paramita* (Vow/Determina-
tion), *Bala Paramita* (Spiritual Power), and *Jnana
Paramita* (Wisdom/ Knowledge).

One who has *bodhichitta* (defined by Maitreya
as "the wish [*chitta*] to become enlightened [*bo-
dhi*] for others") as the primary motivation for
all of one's activities is called a Bodhisattva. It is
sometimes believed that Bodhisattvas are beings
who have "stayed behind" to help others attain
enlightenment, but this is a misunderstanding.
They wish to attain complete enlightenment

(Buddhahood) in order to be of benefit to all sentient beings. Bodhisattvas are not, as is commonly thought, "beings trapped in cyclic existence (*samsara*) who have put off enlightenment to help others." If a Bodhisattva is not enlightened, she cannot help others reach enlightenment.

page 21 For a concise discussion of the stages to awakening, I am indebted to Ken Wilber's *Integral Spirituality*, which cites Daniel P. Brown's study of the great spiritual guides of Buddhism and Hinduism—*The Yoga Sutras* of Patanjali, the *Visuddhimagga* of Buddhaghosha, and the Tibetan *Phyag chen zla ba'i 'od zer* (*Moonbeams of Mahamudra*) by Tashi Namgyal, which describes three stages of evolution on the spiritual path. Paraphrased, they are (1) discipline in committing to the preliminaries of spiritual practice/physical training; (2) a subtle experience of luminosity (ultimate reality) followed by a "dark night of the soul," which is a kind of test, pulling one down again into dualism; and, finally, (3) a breakthrough to non-dual awareness or enlightenment.

"heaven is at hand": A wonderful interpretation of this belief is found in Eckhart Tolle's *A New Earth*.

page 28 *Tonglen*: Tibetan. *Tong* = giving others happiness, *len* = taking away their pain. *Tonglen* is a meditation practice of first taking away another's pain, then giving them happiness. It is also called "Taking Away the Darkness."

page 34 "this passing is all": Craig Arnold, *Made Flesh*. Arnold, a young American poet and professor, came to Japan in the spring of 2009 to work on a book about volcanoes as part of a Creative Artists' Exchange Fellowship from the Japan-U.S. Friendship Commission. On April 27, he went missing on the small volcanic island of Kuchino-erabu-jima, Japan, where he'd gone for a solo hike to explore an active volcano. He never returned to the inn where he was staying. His trail was found near a high cliff, and he was presumed to have died from a fatal fall. He was forty-one years old.

page 36   *Naikan*. Japanese. An aspect of this practice of "inner viewing" is investigating areas in one's life for which one is beholden to others.

page 38   *Prasad*. Sanskrit. Literally, "a gracious gift." An offering, usually a sweet or some other food, blessed by an enlightened being and given to his or her followers.

page 76   *Sadhana*. Sanskrit. Daily spiritual practice, such as meditation, mantra, devotion.

page 86   "it's a good day to live": Osho, *A Sudden Clash of Thunder*.

page 87   "like a blind man": Kagyu Master Jamgon Kongtrul Lodro Thaye.

page 90   "ought to be called Happiness": Raymond Carver, *All of Us: The Collected Poems*.

page 116   *Ehipassiko*. Pali. "Come and see!"

page 125   "supreme, truly perfect enlightenment": R. C. Jamieson, trans., *The Perfection of Wisdom*.

BIBLIOGRAPHY

The following works were gratefully consulted in the preparation
of this book:

Arnold, Craig. *Made Flesh.* Port Townsend, WA: Copper
Canyon, 2008.

Carver, Raymond. *All of Us: The Collected Poems.* New York:
Vintage, 2000.

Cohen, Leonard. *Stranger Music: Selected Poems and Songs.*
New York: Vintage, 1994.

Hafiz. *The Gift.* Translated by Daniel Ladinsky. New York:
Penguin, 1999.

Hirshfield, Jane, ed. *Women in Praise of the Sacred: 43 Centuries
of Spiritual Poetry by Women.* New York: Harper Perennial,
1995.

Jamieson, R. C., trans. *The Perfection of Wisdom.* New York:
Viking Studio, 2000.

Kornfield, Jack. *Your Buddha Nature: Teachings on the Ten
Perfections.* Audiobook. Louisville, CO: Sounds True, 1998.

McNally, Lama Christie. *The Tibetan Book of Meditation.* New
York: Doubleday, 2009.

Osho. *A Sudden Clash of Thunder: Talks on Zen Stories.* New
Delhi: Wisdom Tree, 1977.

Rinchen, Geshe Sonam. *How Karma Works: The Twelve Links
of Dependent Arising.* Translated by Ruth Sonam. Ithaca, NY:
Snow Lion, 2006.

Roach, Geshe Michael. *The Diamond Cutter: The Buddha on

Managing Your Business and Your Life. New York: Doubleday, 2000.

——— and Christie McNally. *The Essential Yoga Sutra: Ancient Wisdom for Your Yoga*. New York: Doubleday, 2005.

Rumi, Jalal Al-Din. *The Illuminated Rumi*. Translated by Coleman Barks. New York: Broadway Books, 2000.

Snyder, Gary. *Turtle Island*. New York: New Directions, 1969.

Tarthang Tulku. *Skillful Means: Patterns for Success*. Oakland, CA: Dharma Publishing, 1991.

Tolle, Eckhart. *A New Earth*. New York: Plume, 2006.

Wilber, Ken. *Integral Spirituality: A Startling New Role for Religion in the Modern and Postmodern World*. Boston: Shambhala, 2007.